Better Mental Health

And Fitness

By

Nicole Carter

Contents

Better Mental Health And Fitness

By Nicole Carter

Succinct and easy to read, expert motivation and advice on how to use fitness and healthy nutrition, as complementary therapy to improve your mental health and fitness.

This guide will help you to make healthier nutrition and activity choices, which may help to alter your brain and body chemistry in a positive way. This book explains how to utilise your body's natural Fight-or-flight response chemicals, more effectively, by using moderate exercise and good nutrition.

This may alleviate some of the symptoms of stress, depression and anxiety, at the same time as improving your physical fitness.

Ask your Doctor first about any changes you are planning to make to your current lifestyle, and if you want to start a new fitness and nutrition program. Please use this book as complementary therapy, in conjunction with your doctor's advice and prescriptions. This book is packed with interesting and useful information, to help you set realistic long-term goals for your nutrition and fitness.

Start your journey towards improving your mental health and physical health today!!

Introduction

The information in this guide, has been researched and gathered by myself, from various reliable sources online (such as the National Health Service Choices website), and from relevant books, after many years of fitness training for my personal health, and training other people. My qualifications include nutrition advice, as well as fitness testing, and instruction.

I studied my SVQ Level 2 at Stevenson College in 2004-2005, and gained my instructor qualifications for exercise to music, circuits and gym. I then got my Level 3 personal trainer qualification with Premier Global NASM in 2005.

I have had further training from the Nutrition and Weight Management Centre in 2005, while I was working at a private health club in Edinburgh, as a fitness class instructor and personal trainer.

I have worked as an outdoor activities instructor, near Dunoon on the West coast of Scotland, and near Hemsby in Norfolk, England. I've also worked with elderly and disabled people as a chair-based exercise class instructor, and activities organiser in a nursing home.

Through trial and error, I have found that many of the symptoms of my Bi-polar mental health disorder, have been reasonably alleviated, by using fitness and good nutrition as a complement to my prescribed medication.

This Guide is meant as complementary therapy advice, to be used in conjunction with your Doctor's advice and prescriptions, not as a substitute to medication and NHS mental health services.

Yes, I have not always practiced what I preach hence me saying "Through trial and error" at the beginning of the previous paragraph. Having a mental health condition is a complex issue, and I personally still struggle at times; however, it is through the good and the bad experiences I have had over the years, that I have realised how getting into good positive routines, self-care, openness and honesty with people I know well and trust, as well as medication, and using the mental health services as often as I need to, all helps me a great deal.

I personally have realised that pushing myself to "go further" sometimes, helps me to put life's other challenges into perspective.

As a child growing up in a suburban area, I climbed trees, went swimming and played other types of sport with my friends and family.

I believe very strongly that, as a child is growing and developing, if they are able to utilise both sides of their body by doing monitored sports such as climbing, swimming and balancing games to enhance the proprioceptive response (balance and core response), this can help their brain develop more healthily.

This will also mean they may be better able to process the natural Fight-or-flight hormones and neurotransmitters more effectively, which may also help to reduce stress, depression and anxiety.

This book explains why doing regular moderate intensity fitness activities and sports, combined with eating regular healthy nutrition, getting enough water hydration intake, and getting enough rest, can be beneficial for both children and adults; because this may help to alter brain and body chemistry in a positive way, by enabling the natural Fight-or-flight response chemicals, to be processed more efficiently by the brain and body.

Your decision to read this guide is an indication that you are looking for answers and / or help to improve your life, you have made that choice, you have made that pro-active move to change what you don't like. Please be proud of yourself and give yourself the recognition you deserve.

Everything in moderation! Yes, that includes cream buns, pizza, crisps and chocolate, because it is possible that if you deny yourself these treats totally, some people are more likely to binge on them. Consider these as a weekend treat rather than eating them every day.

Eat slowly, savour your food. Food is one of life's great pleasures, NOT your enemy!

Many people would see an immediate improvement in how they look and feel, if they simply improved their posture by standing up straighter, putting their chin and shoulders into a neutral position and, not holding-in their abs, but engaging their core muscles.

An easy, sensible way to start being more active, is to think of ways you could incorporate exercise into your daily routine, for example, getting off the bus a few stops early so you can walk some of the way to work or college; Using the stairs instead of the lift or escalator; Instead of taking the car to the shops, walk there and take the bus back with your shopping more often, rather than getting your shopping all in one go.

You could try sitting on a Swiss Ball to watch TV rather than sitting on the sofa or desk chair. This will be an "invisible workout" for your core muscles. Get the right size of ball for your height, sit with good posture, knees at 90 degrees and feet flat on the ground.

If you are interested in finding out even more about fitness and nutrition and are curious to know why it is so important, then please read on. At the end of each section there is a checklist for you to read and write down in a notepad, to help you remember the main points and set goals.

At the end of the book there are templates for you to re-write a brief food, mood and energy diary for 5 days, in a notepad, to help you see where you could make changes, and modify your activity levels and nutrition intake.

There is also a template for you to write down your goals for nutrition and fitness, in your notepad.

I hope you find this guide useful and enjoy reading it. You should be proud of yourself for taking an interest in healthy nutrition and fitness, good luck, believe in yourself, and HAVE FUN with your training!

Nicole Carter

Your Metabolism is the set of chemical reactions that happen in all living organisms (including humans) to maintain life. These processes allow organisms to grow and reproduce, maintain their structures and respond to their environments. Metabolism is usually divided into two categories:

Catabolism breaks down food to harvest energy.

Anabolism uses that energy to construct essential components of body cells, such as proteins and nucleic acids, for body cell maintenance and repair.

Basal and Resting Metabolic rates are different for each person, and relative to the amount of food consumed, and their exercise levels.

Both can influence how quickly an individual processes energy input (food), and their energy levels for motivation to adhere to activity.

Cardiovascular training, and especially using weights to train your muscles, will help your metabolic rates become more efficient at burning calories and fat, even when resting; hence needing to eat according to your training level.

After a long period of an unchanged routine in exercise level, and food intake, your metabolic rates can plateau, so they may need re-adjusted to enhance performance for exercise, and to increase energy levels.

For someone who has trained a lot in exercise and sport, at school for example, but then is unable to train through injury, or from studying or working full-time, it is possible that their hunger levels will stay the same, but due to inability to work off the calories by exercising, they can put on weight.

It is important that after a hiatus in your training, that you keep positive and feel confident that you will get back on track **when you are ready**.

DON'T give yourself a hard time to the point that it stops you from resuming your activities.

Most people who have done exercise in the past at school for example, will still have muscle memory, and that means they can re-engage their body's ability to move actively, if they follow a slow, sensible progressive plan.

Physical health and mental health are intrinsically co-existent, so after asking your doctor's advice, and seeking the appropriate recommended assistance, keep focused and just know that you are worth being good to yourself, and be kind to yourself.

Worry can be debilitating so harness all that positivity you felt before, to get you back to feeling good again. You CAN do it!!

Nutrition Guidelines

Healthy nutrition and cold-water hydration every 2 and a ½ to 3 hours during the day, (or waking hours if you work shifts), encourages the body to have the energy to start and maintain a progressive exercise program. By maintaining good physical health, it is possible your mental health will improve too.

This nutrition routine when included with regular moderate intensity activity, is likely to encourage the body to process these key Fight-or-flight hormones and neurotransmitters (among many others), more effectively: Serotonin, adrenaline, dopamine, endorphins and cortisol;

This may help to alleviate some of the symptoms of stress, anxiety and depression.

Eating and drinking a glass of cold water every 2 and a ½ to 3 hours, during waking hours, also helps you to maintain your concentration levels for work and studying and balances your mood and metabolic rates. This may also help to reduce fatigue, anxiety, headaches, stress and mild depression.

Cortisol: Eating regularly prevents an energy low and reduces the amount of the stress steroid hormone cortisol, which is produced by the body to retain calories and fat, when you have a diet that is too low in calories and "good" fats.

Long-term low-calorie diets tend not to work because of this reaction. Initially they will make you lose weight, but then you may feel fatigued, and end up binging on high calorie foods, to compensate for your body's low level of blood-glucose from eating too little.

According to the First Aid courses training I've done, hunger and low blood-glucose can also cause anger, stress, anxiety and belligerence.

Regular eating will help to rebalance your metabolic rates, and maintain energy and concentration levels, which will make you feel like being more active.

Even if you are not that active, eating healthily every 2 and a ½ to 3 hours, and keeping hydrated with water, will make sure you keep feeling good mentally and physically, and will mean you may be more likely to weigh a sensible weight for your height, within a relatively short period of time after starting this kind of energising eating plan, as you will feel more like being active.

Take slow, small logical steps back to strength. Try to have 3 main meals, plus a mid-morning snack, mid-afternoon snack, and a light supper 2 hours before bed.

Eating and drinking too soon before bed can cause acid reflux, and disturbed sleep but eating a supper at the right time, may help you sleep better.

For your main meals and two snacks, include protein from any of these sources: Fish or meat or poultry or vegetarian / vegan alternatives. Also include low to medium Glycemic Index (GI) carbohydrates and vegetables, in at least two of your main meals.

Examples of protein sources and GI carbohydrates are given on the next few pages.

Water intake, main meals and snacks in-between meals should be in quantities relative to your exercise training levels. With each meal and snack, remember to drink at least a small to medium sized glass of cold tap water.

Snack and supper ideas

Examples of mid-morning and mid-afternoon snacks or supper, you could choose from:

1 snack or supper if you do moderate exercise such as the equivalent of a 5k brisk walk or jog 2-4 times a week, or a 10k brisk walk or jog 1-2 times a week;

*A small bowl of soup or

*2 oatcakes or corncakes, spread thinly with butter, with thin slices of cheddar cheese, or 2 teaspoons of cottage cheese, or pate or houmous or nut butter + slices of cucumber or tomato. Or

*A full fat dairy yogurt + a piece of fruit or

*A small bowl of cereal with full fat milk or

*One small, cooked chicken breast fillet or

*2 peeled hard-boiled eggs or

*2 scrambled eggs or

*Raw vegetable crudité with ½ a tub of houmous or

*Two 1-inch cubes of cheese or

*A slice of wholemeal toast with butter, or nut butter, or cottage cheese or

*5 Falafel

For someone who is sedentary (mostly inactive) a mid-morning or mid-afternoon snack or supper could be:

*A small piece of fruit or

*A palmful of mixed dried fruit & unsalted nuts & seeds or

*A palmful of fresh berries or

*An oatcake or corncake with a thin layer of low fat spread or

*A low-fat yogurt or

*Raw vegetables crudité or

*Two small, thin slices of cooked meat or

*A 1-inch cube of cheese or

*3 teaspoons of nut butter or cottage cheese or

*2 Falafel

Another option for a light supper could be a bowl of unsweetened puffed rice, or unsweetened puffed wheat (any unsweetened cereal) with soya, or almond, or oat, or rice milk, if you are vegan or vegetarian; or cow's or goat's milk.

Dairy milk and other dairy products contain a lot of tryptophan, which helps the body produce melatonin, which in turn helps you to sleep.

Another idea for a healthy supper for a moderately active person, is a slice of wholegrain toast with a thin spread of unsalted butter, or nut butter, or cottage cheese. Eating and drinking too soon before going to bed may cause disturbed sleep however, eating a light supper 2 hours before going to bed, may help you sleep better and feel more energised in the morning.

Bodybuilders and other people who regularly do strenuous exercise, will need to eat a lot more for their main meals and snacks. There are comprehensive sports nutrition books you can buy to find out more.

It would also be beneficial to remember that small to moderate amounts of "good" cholesterol fat from food, helps the body to produce the steroid hormones testosterone and oestrogen, which is essential to maintain muscle mass and regulate your mood.

Calculate your daily calorie requirements

Your daily calorie needs will depend on your genetics, age, weight, body composition, your daily activity level and your training program.

Your Basal Metabolic Rate (BMR) is the number of calories you burn at rest (to keep your heart beating, your lungs breathing, to maintain your body temperature etc).   It accounts for 60-75% of the calories you burn daily.

It is possible to estimate the number of calories you need daily, from your body weight (in Kilograms), and your level of daily physical activity, using this calculation I adapted from trainer and author Anita Bean's books:

Step 1: Estimate your Basal Metabolic Rate (BMR): BMR uses 23 calories for every Kg of a sedentary person's bodyweight, and 24 calories per Kg of an active person's bodyweight:

Sedentary people: BMR = weight in Kg x 23

Active people: BMR = weight in Kg x 24

Step 2: Work out your Physical Activity Level (PAL): This is the ratio of your overall daily energy expenditure to your BMR – a rough measure of your lifestyle activity:

*Mostly inactive or sedentary (mainly sitting): PAL = 1.2

*Fairly active (walking / exercise 1-2 times a week): PAL = 1.3

*Moderately active (exercise 2-3 times a week): PAL = 1.4

*Active (exercise hard more than 3 times a week): PAL = 1.5

*Very active (exercise hard daily): PAL = 1.7

Step 3: BMR x PAL = your approximate daily calories needs to maintain your current weight. The result you get from this calculation, gives you an approximation of your daily calories requirement to **maintain** your current weight.

REMEMBER: REST IS VERY IMPORTANT TOO, so exercising hard every day is **not** recommended for a prolonged period of time.

Use the **Food, Mood and Energy Diary** templates at the end of the book, to briefly detail all food, hydration, mood and energy levels throughout the day, to give you a better idea as to what changes or modifications you could make to your daily nutrition intake, and plan how you can become more energised in the long-term.

Try writing down in a notepad EVERYTHING you eat and drink, your mood, your energy levels and activities, in the time slot boxes HONESTLY, every day for 1 week.

If you find you have a specific food intolerance speak to your Doctor. Food intolerances are very common, there are many supermarkets and health food shops that sell healthy, tasty alternatives.

Fibre: Vegetables & fruit contain varying proportions of vitamins, provitamins and some contain carbohydrates. Vegetables also contain a great variety of other phytochemicals (plant-based natural chemicals); some of which may have antioxidant, antibacterial, antifungal, antiviral and cancer fighting properties.

Most vegetables contain fibre, which is important for gut health and regular bowel functions.

Vegetables and fruit also contain important nutrients necessary for healthy hair, and skin as well.

Diets containing recommended amounts of fruits and vegetables, may help lower the risk of heart-diseases, type 2 diabetes and prevent bone-density loss.

The potassium provided by both fruits and vegetables, may help prevent the formation of kidney stones.

Health professionals recommend you have 3 different vegetables, of different colours every day, either rinsed and eaten raw or cooked until slightly al dente to retain all the nutrients.

How you cook vegetables can really affect their taste, texture and nutrient level.

Over-cooked vegetables don't taste as good, and don't have the same amount of nutrients as vegetables that are washed and eaten raw, or that are steamed, roasted or lightly boiled until slightly al-dente. Steamed, roasted or boiled vegetables that are cooked for the recommended amount of time, taste great and will give you lots of natural fibre, vitamins and minerals.

Home-cooked food tastes so much better because you can adapt recipes to suit your individual tastes.

Most pre-prepared foods have a lot of extra salt and other additives that you wouldn't normally use at home, cooking your own food is enjoyable too.

Even if you are cooking for just yourself and money is tight, you can cook your own healthy, nutritious meals for a lot less than you would pay for ready meals. You can cook extra to freeze or have the following day, which is more economical and saves time. There are lots of great easy to follow recipe books available.

Preparing a lunch to take to work or college every day is a great idea too, and a lot cheaper.

When I've struggled with my own mental health, I have eaten ready-meals or takeaways, but only at times when I've been unable to cook my own meals from fresh ingredients. You need to eat to keep your strength up, do what feels right for you.

The Glycemic Index (GI) is a measure of the effects of carbohydrates on blood-sugar levels. Carbohydrates that break down quickly during digestion and release glucose rapidly into the bloodstream, have a high GI; Carbohydrates that break down more slowly, releasing glucose more gradually into the bloodstream, have a low GI.

A low GI food will release glucose more slowly and steadily, which leads to more suitable blood-glucose readings after each meal, and a regular more even level of energy throughout the day.

A high GI food causes a more rapid rise in blood-glucose levels, and may be suitable for energy recovery after exercise, or for a person experiencing hypoglycemia (low blood-glucose), but they should be limited in the diet as they induce an energy "spike", followed quickly by an energy dip.

Please refer to the table on the next page and add any other foods you've found that are in each GI range. Remember to limit your intake of the foods in the High GI range.

Table of examples from the Glycemic Index

Glycemic Level	GI Range	Examples
Low GI	55 or less	Most fruits, most vegetables, legumes / pulses, nuts, seeds, oats, corn cakes, fructose, brown rice, unsweetened dairy products, whole-wheat pasta, whole-wheat tortilla.
Medium GI	56 – 59	Some fruits, basmati rice, sweet potato, sucrose, dried fruit, couscous, pitta bread.
High GI	70+	Refined processed products: e.g. White bread, white rice, sweetened breakfast cereals, glucose, maltose, baked potatoes, rice cakes.

How much protein is enough?

Health professionals suggest that most people should consume 0.8g of protein per Kg of your own current bodyweight, per day. In practical terms, eating a moderate amount of protein, in one or two meals every day, should give you all the protein you need. Endurance athletes and bodybuilders will need to tailor their real-food-protein intake according to their energy expenditure.

Be wary of protein and whey shakes, they often contain harmful amounts of unnecessary ingredients (like synthetic vitamins and minerals) and can possibly cause kidney and liver problems.

The biggest body builders I've ever met include full-fat milk, full-fat yoghurt and cheese in their high protein diet, they also eat LOTS of fresh vegetables, some fruit AND carbohydrates!!!

A proper balanced diet without supplements is ideal to keep you healthy, fit and avoid injury and illness. Whey powder is a by-product of the cheese-making industry, so why not just enjoy the varied delicious cheeses you can buy, if you are able to.

It is recommended that you eat **one or two servings** of real-food-protein **every day,** from both plant and animal sources.

Here are some examples of one serving, about the size of a standard pack of playing cards:

*70g boneless meat (e.g. lean beef, lamb or pork)

*70g boneless poultry (e.g. 1 chicken, duck or turkey breast)

*70g or 1 fillet of fish (e.g. salmon, sardines or tuna, haddock, mackerel)

*2 medium eggs

*85g mix of seeds (e.g. linseeds, sunflower seeds or pumpkin seeds), and nuts (e.g. almonds, pine nuts, Brazil nuts or walnuts) e.g. in a nut roast, or nut burgers, or nut butter.

*85g mix of beans and pulses (e.g. pinto beans, butter beans, red lentils, chickpeas, soya beans, green lentils, kidney beans)

*85g of Myco-protein or soya protein (e.g. Quorn, tofu, Textured Vegetable Protein)

Which nutrients are best for providing energy?

Muscles use two main fuels - carbohydrate and fat. Carbohydrates provide rapidly available energy and are therefore the most important energy source for short, intense exercise like sprinting. When exercising at full capacity, the energy requirement is so great and needed so quickly, that only carbohydrates can produce energy fast enough.

The body stores limited amounts of carbohydrates - enough for approximately 20 to 30 minutes of moderate exercise. After this, if fat cannot be converted to energy during high intensity exercise, the body becomes fatigued.

The body can use fat for supplying energy during longer periods of exercise at a more moderate pace.

For those people exercising to help them lose excess body-fat, it's best to exercise for longer periods at a moderate level to burn fat, e.g. cycling, swimming or aqua aerobics or brisk walking or jogging for longer than 30 minutes. Remember to eat according to your activity level to keep your energy levels good and keep you motivated.

Whatever the intensity of the exercise, some carbohydrates are always used, and it's important to replenish stores before the next session.

It is best to top up carbohydrates straight after exercising, by eating a piece of fruit for example, or drinking a fruit juice plus water mix, and eating a full balanced meal within an hour of exercising.

A good alternative to standard energy drinks is a mixture of: Rice milk for quick acting high GI carbohydrate energy, plus soya or almond milk for protein, plus oat milk for slow-release low GI carbohydrate energy.

Try this by getting a sports water bottle, and mixing your own energy drink, and remember to keep it in the fridge when you are not using it. High sugar high GI energy drinks can give you that energy high, but it's quickly followed by an energy low, so they aren't ideal for during training.

Kick-start your metabolism by eating a good, hearty breakfast, to set you up for the day and give you energy to work, study etc.

Carbohydrates: Health professionals advise that most people should have approximately 1/3 of their balanced daily nutrition intake, from varied complex carbohydrates (low to medium Glycemic Index starchy foods); examples include:

Wholegrain pasta, wholegrain bread, brown rice, potatoes, bulgur wheat, couscous, barley, noodles, oats and other unrefined grains, plantains and low-sugar cereals. Make sure you serve one of these with vegetables and protein in two of your main meals, every day. Many complex carbohydrates are also a good source of fibre.

Essential Fatty Acids or EFAs, are fatty-acids that humans and other animals must ingest because the body requires them for good health, but cannot make them all by itself. The term "essential fatty acid" refers to fatty acids required for biological processes, and not those that only act as fuel.

Examples of sources of Omega 3 and 6 EFA's are fish and shellfish, flaxseed (linseed) oil, soya oil, canola oil, dark green leafy vegetables and most unsalted nuts and seeds. Do your own research into how to get the best forms of these nutrients to suit you.

Research suggests that moderate intakes of fish and omega-3 fatty acids, are linked to decreased rates of major depression, and can improve the symptoms of high blood pressure and certain types of arthritis, due to its anti-inflammatory qualities.

Omega 3 fatty acids are important for enzymatic pathways required to metabolise polyunsaturated fatty acids.

Correlations have been found between depression and low levels of omega-3 fatty acids, and treatment with omega-3 supplementation has shown benefit for depression, as well as other mood disorders. Of course, eating properly cooked fish once or twice a week, is even better than taking a supplement.

Please discuss with your doctor before taking any supplements during pregnancy, if you are breastfeeding or on any medication.

High-density lipoprotein (HDL) also known as "Good" Cholesterol, is one of the five major groups of lipoproteins, which enable lipids like cholesterol and triglycerides, to be transported within the water-based bloodstream. Studies have shown that high concentrations of HDL, have protective value against cardiovascular diseases such as ischemic stroke and heart attacks.

Low concentrations of HDL increase the risk for atherosclerotic diseases (artery wall thickening with fatty deposits).

Delivery of HDL cholesterol to adrenals, ovaries, and testes is important for the synthesis of steroid hormones: Oestrogen and testosterone.

Eating a regular balanced nutrition intake, including moderate amounts of unsalted nuts, seeds and fresh fish, stopping smoking, reducing alcohol intake, moderate exercise, and maintaining the correct body-fat % for your age, all help to increase HDL levels in the body.

Low Density Lipoprotein (LDL) is one of the five major groups of lipoproteins that enable transport of cholesterol within the water-based bloodstream.

Studies have shown that higher levels of type-B LDL particles (as opposed to type-A LDL particles) can cause health problems and cardiovascular disease; they are often informally called the "Bad cholesterol" particles.

Reducing visceral fat around the organs with moderate exercise, plus eating a balanced nutrition intake, with recommended amounts of vegetables and fruit, stopping smoking, and reducing your alcohol intake, can help to lower LDL levels.

Adipose tissue (Body-fat) is loose connective tissue composed of adipocytes. It is technically composed of roughly only 80% fat; Fat in its solitary state exists in the liver and muscles. The main role of adipose tissue is to store energy in the form of lipids, although it also cushions and insulates the body. The brain is comprised of a high percentage of lipid fats, so we need a certain amount of various fats and oils in our nutrition intake.

Hydrogenated fats and Trans fats are not recommended, check your food labels.

Adipose tissue has in recent years been recognised as a **major essential endocrine organ,** as it produces hormones such as leptin (which controls hunger levels), resistin (which is an indicator for obesity-related Type 2 Diabetes), and the cytokine TNFα (which signals to other cells to deal with inflammation and disease).

Excess adipose tissue can affect other organ systems of the body, and may lead to disease. Obesity or being overweight does not depend on body weight, but on the amount of body-fat.

The Body Mass Index (or BMI) is an inaccurate method of determining your actual body composition, as it only uses your age, weight and height to calculate the result.

Your BMI could be an inaccurate gauge of your weight, because you could have more muscle than someone who is the same weight, height and age as you. Body composition analysis devices are a much better way of telling you how much water, fat and muscle you have, although they are expensive.

Many body builders are classed as "obese" according to their BMI, which shows how inaccurate BMI can be. My advice is - "DITCH THE SCALES!!" You can buy skin-fold calipers, they are much more reliable with their result, and not expensive.

Measuring yourself around the chest, waist, thighs, arms and hips, may also help you to gauge your progress with fat loss, or fat gain, increased muscle-mass and increased fitness. Write the measurements down in a 6-weekly chart.

Be aware though, that increased muscle-mass from regular weightlifting and core-stabiliser training, can affect these measurements. Many women can be prone to having a stronger sturdier core and waist measurement, because they are capable of becoming pregnant, so their abdomens are naturally going to be bigger, even if they are not pregnant.

Please check out the body-fat percentages for your age-range on the next page.

Table of body-fat percentages

Women: Aged	Underfat	Healthy range	Overfat	Obese
20 > 40	Under 21%	**21 – 33%**	33 – 39%	Over 39%
41 > 60	Under 23%	**23 – 35%**	35 – 40%	Over 40%
61 > 79	Under 24%	**24 – 36%**	36 – 42%	Over 42%
Men: Aged	Underfat	Healthy range	Overfat	Obese
20 > 40	Under 8%	**8 – 19%**	19 – 25%	Over 25%
41 > 60	Under 11%	**11 – 22%**	22 – 27%	Over 27%
61 > 79	Under 13%	**13 – 25%**	25 – 30%	Over 30%

The benefits of unsalted nuts and seeds

Several studies have revealed that people who consume unsalted nuts and seeds regularly are less likely to suffer from Coronary Heart Disease (CHD). Nuts were first linked to protection against CHD in 1993.

Since then, many clinical trials have found that consumption of various unsalted nuts and seeds such as almonds, Brazil nuts, hazelnuts, pine nuts, linseeds, sunflower seeds, pumpkin seeds, cashews and walnuts etc. can lower Low Density Lipoprotein cholesterol concentrations. Unsalted nuts and seeds apparently contain various substances thought to have cardio-protective effects, and scientists believe that their Omega 3 fatty acids are partly responsible for this response observed in clinical trials.

In addition to having cardio-protective effects, unsalted nuts and seeds generally are very low on the Glycemic Index (GI).

Dietitians frequently recommend unsalted nuts and seeds, to be included in diets prescribed for patients with insulin resistance problems, such as diabetes mellitus type 2. One study found that people who eat unsalted nuts and seeds, live two to three years longer than those who do not. However, this may be because people who eat unsalted nuts and seeds tend to eat less junk food.

Unsalted nuts and seeds also contain the essential fatty acids linoleic and linolenic acids and the fats in nuts are mostly unsaturated fats, including mono-unsaturated fats, which are deemed to be healthier than the saturated fats from meat.

Recent studies show that a very small amount of saturated fats from meat, can actually be a beneficial addition to your food intake, if you can eat them.

Many unsalted nuts and seeds are good sources of vitamins E and B_2, and are rich in protein, folate, fibre, and essential minerals such as magnesium, phosphorus, potassium, copper, and selenium. Nuts and seeds are most healthy in their raw unsalted form. The reason is that up to 15% of the healthy oils that naturally occur in nuts are lost during the roasting process.

Although initial studies suggested that antioxidants might promote health, later large clinical trials did not detect any benefit, and suggested instead that excess consumption is harmful.

As I said before, **everything in moderation**! Try replacing some of your crisps and sweets with raw unsalted nuts and seeds, if you already know you can. If you have an allergy to these, there are other good snack options to choose from; please refer to the previous section in the Nutrition Guidelines.

Fat soluble vitamins A, D, E, K

Fat-soluble vitamins include the vitamins A, D, E and K. They are essential for general good health, the daily repair of body cells and efficient functioning of body organs.

As the name suggests, they're carried into the body by fats from your food intake, which is why certain fats are necessary in your diet.

A deficiency of fat-soluble vitamins may occur in people with poor nutrition intake, or those suffering from long-term conditions that affect their ability to absorb fats from the intestine.

Balanced, varied nutrition intake in quantities relative to your exercise level will provide most people with enough of these vitamins, and it is **NOT** necessary to take specific supplements unless advised by your doctor. A very useful book to find real-food sources of various vitamins and minerals is The Vitamin and Mineral Counter by Jody Vassallo.

Phospholipids; necessary components of all the body's cell membranes including brain cells. These membranes form a continuous barrier around cells. Lipid bi-layer membranes, are the barriers that keep ions, proteins and other molecules where they are needed, and prevent them from diffusing into areas where they should not be.

According to archaeologists' research, our hunter-gatherer ancestors evolved mostly on a diet of animal offal, nuts, seeds, berries, tubers, fish and shellfish.

Fish, shellfish nuts and seeds contain essential fatty acids, and offal, such as in liver pate and haggis, contain phospholipids, which are deemed a useful part of your nutrition intake (if you can eat them), as we still need these nutrients, to maintain the health of our brain and body cells.

I often have a piece of fruit and 2 slices of wholemeal toast, or a wholemeal wrap, with pate, or houmous, or peanut butter for breakfast, and I make sure I include haggis or blackpudding in one or two balanced meals, every month.

Salt, MSG, sugar & artificial sweeteners

Too much salt in your food means you are not getting the full flavour of the food you are eating, try to retrain your tastebuds to need less salt as it can increase blood pressure, and causes many other health problems.

MSG (Mono-sodium-glutamate) is an artificial high sodium-based flavor enhancer for savoury foods. Check your food labels to see if what you are buying contains MSG and avoid products that contain it.

There is a lot of evidence to suggest that artificial sweeteners are not good for you. There are a few on the market now that are "natural plant-based" sweeteners, however, try to retrain your tastebuds to need less sweet flavours too, and you will find that you can taste the actual food rather than just the sweetness.

Everyone knows what too much sugar does to your body and how it can rot teeth, increase your fat levels, and in the long term may cause type 2 diabetes.

How to utilise the Fight-or-flight stress response

Adrenaline is a hormone and a neurotransmitter. It increases heart rate, constricts blood vessels, dilates air passages and participates in the Fight-or-flight response of the nervous system, i.e. The Survival Instinct.

"Adrenaline addict" is a term used to describe somebody who appears to be addicted to adrenaline and such a person is sometimes described as getting a "high" from life.

Adrenaline addicts appear to favour stressful activities, as the body releases adrenaline as a stress response to extreme sports for example.

Doing this may result in physical harm because of the potential danger.

Whether or not the positive response is caused specifically by adrenaline, is difficult to determine, as endorphins are also released during the Fight-or-flight response to such activities.

Building up gradually and sensibly to moderate levels of regular exercise, will also give you an adrenaline "rush" a natural high, and may help to reduce the anxiety caused when you get that Fight-or-flight response from stressful situations at work, home or college etc;

Keeping active, hydrated, eating well and getting enough rest, may help to alter your brain and body chemistry in a positive way, by processing the Fight-or-flight response chemicals more efficiently.

Modern life is very different to how we lived as hunter-gatherers; many people are more "sedentary" which means they don't exercise very often.

Our ancestors would have been very active hunting and gathering food when they could, they also had to be fit to run or fight in dangerous situations; this is what the "Fight-or-flight" response is for, it keeps you alert, and able to make split-second decisions, to keep you alive.

These days anxiety, stress and depression may be indications that many people aren't as active as they could be, or not eating the right foods for their level of activity.

Many mental health conditions seem to be connected to the natural prehistoric response mechanism of Fight-or-flight, the body and brain's requirements to be able to cope with stress or danger, and to process the hormones and neurotransmitters detailed in this book, as well as many others.

Over the years I have personally realised that in order to keep mentally well, I have to eat healthily regularly throughout the day, keep hydrated with water, make sure I get enough **sleep,** keep taking my Bipolar medication and keep moderately active.

During more serious training, I rest for 2 weeks from my training program every 3 months, to allow my body to recover and muscle tissue to repair, build and tone. Relaxation time is very important too, so I try to schedule in quality "Me time" as regularly as I need to.

Endorphins ("endogenous morphine") are neurotransmitters (chemical messengers). They are produced during exercise, excitement, feelings of love and consumption of spicy food, to give a feeling of well-being.

They are produced by the pituitary gland (the major endocrine gland that is important in controlling growth and development), and in the hypothalamus (section of the brain responsible for the production of many of the body's essential hormones).

The term endorphin rush has been adopted in popular speech, to refer to feelings of exhilaration brought on by physical exertion, supposedly due to the influence of endorphins. When a nerve impulse reaches the spinal cord, endorphins are released which prevent nerve cells from releasing more pain signals.

Serotonin is a neurotransmitter. Biochemically derived from tryptophan, serotonin is primarily found in the Gastro-Intestinal tract, blood platelets and in the Central Nervous System of humans.

It is thought to be a contributor to feelings of wellbeing; therefore, it is also known as a "Happiness Hormone" despite not being a hormone.

Approximately 80 percent of the human body's total serotonin is in cells in the gut, where it is used to regulate intestinal movements.

Serotonin also has roles in regulation of mood, appetite, sleep, as well as muscle contraction and in some cognitive functions, including in memory and learning.

Balance of serotonin at synapses in the brain, is thought to be a major action of several classes of pharmacological anti-depressant and anti-psychotic medications.

Synapses are junctions between two nerve cells, consisting of a minute gap across which, impulses pass by diffusion of neurotransmitters such as serotonin.

Serotonin levels can also be affected by your nutrition intake, however, do please follow your Dr's advice to keep well.

Research suggests eating a diet rich in carbohydrates, and low in protein will increase serotonin by secreting insulin, however, increasing insulin for a long period may trigger the onset of insulin resistance, obesity, type 2 diabetes and therefore eventually lower serotonin levels.

A sensible varied, balanced nutrition intake containing protein, carbohydrates, vegetables and fruit, as mentioned before, is recommended.

The benefits of Tryptophan

Tryptophan is an essential amino acid. This means that it cannot be synthesised by the body, and therefore must be part of our nutrition intake. Healthy real-food sources of amino acids, including tryptophan, act as building blocks for cell repair in our bodies.

Tryptophan functions as a biochemical precursor for Serotonin. Serotonin, in turn, can be converted to melatonin (a neurohormone which assists sleep) as explained before.

Muscles use many of the amino acids except tryptophan, allowing some people to have more serotonin than others, unless that person also does muscle training. Most foods contain varying amounts of tryptophan.

Dopamine is a precursor to adrenaline. Dopamine has many functions in the brain, including important roles in behavior and cognition, voluntary movement, motivation, inhibition of prolactin production (involved in lactation), sleep, mood, attention, working memory, and learning; Dopamine is essential for feeling "reward" from eating, drinking, exercising, and bodily functions etc. which means you are more likely to do something again that gives you that good feeling of reward.

Checklist 1: Re-write this table and tick each box once you have read the contents, to make sure you understand the main points of this section and to help you set goals.

	Ask your doctor before you start any new fitness and nutrition routine.
	Make sure you eat every 2 ½ to 3 hours during waking hours, and make sure you drink water every 2 ½ to 3 hours during waking hours, tapering off before bedtime.
	Eat healthy, low-sugar, unsalted snacks and your 3 main balanced meals every day. Keep treats for the weekend.
	1/3 intake of low to medium Glycemic Index carbohydrates.
	Calculate how much protein you need according to your activity levels.
	Cook your vegetables until slightly al dente or eat certain vegetables raw after rinsing them. Eat 2 pieces of fruit and 3 different vegetables daily. Include unsalted nuts, seeds, fish & a little "Good fats & oils" in your balanced nutrition, if you can.
	Don't go by normal scales weight or BMI, get your body-fat % checked at your local gym or use skinfold calipers.

Guidelines for enjoyable exercise:

Don't play sport to get fit,

get fit to play sport!!

When starting a new exercise routine or sport, always seek advice from a qualified, insured instructor or physiotherapist for induction of new equipment, the correct level of fitness program for you and the correct techniques.

Start gradually and train to increase long-term goals progressively over time, eating real-food calories using balanced, healthy, varied, low to medium Glycemic Index foods and healthy hydration, according to your daily training calories expenditure.

This will ensure that you feel motivated for doing activity, through increased energy levels, which therefore encourages adherence.

ALWAYS ask your doctor for their advice before you start any new fitness and nutrition program.

For a simple "invisible workout" you could try sitting on a Swiss Ball instead of the sofa to watch TV for 15-20 minutes 3-4 times a week.

Get the right size of ball for your height, sit with good posture, knees at 90 degrees and your feet flat on the ground. It's amazing how effective this is for training your core muscles (the muscles around your back and abdomen).

Swiss Ball size guide:

"Sizes based upon height are approximate. If you are in between (for instance, you stand between 5′ 5″ and 5′ 6″ tall) you could opt to go either way. Consider your other body characteristics and how you plan to use the ball.

If you are 5′ 5″ and weigh 240 lbs, you should probably use a 65 cm ball.

On the other hand, if you are 5′ 5″, but have very short legs, you might prefer a 55 cm ball.

If you intend to exercise while lying on your back, the smaller ball would work better.

If you are not sure, it is safer to choose the larger size. You always have the option of inflating the ball less. Make sure you are sitting with your knees at 90 degrees."

Your height	Ball height	Ball size
Up to 4'10" (145cm)	18 inches (45cm)	Small
4'8" to 5'5" (140 - 165cm)	22 inches (55cm)	Medium
5'6" to 6'0" (165 - 185cm)	26 inches (65cm)	Large
6'0" to 6'5" (185 - 195cm)	30 inches (75cm)	Extra Large
Over 6'5" (195cm)	33 inches (85cm)	Extra Extra Large

Excerpt and table adapted from SwissBall.com

What powers your muscles?

Muscles are predominately powered when your body processes the fats, protein and carbohydrates from your nutrition intake. Muscle atrophy is defined as a decrease in the mass of the muscle; it can be a partial or complete wasting away of muscle. When a muscle atrophies, this leads to muscle weakness since the ability to exert force is related to muscle mass.

Starvation eventually leads to muscle atrophy, as does too little food intake when training a lot as the body starts to get its protein requirements from your own muscles, this is a process called ketosis and can be dangerous in certain circumstances, such for people with an eating disorder or extreme low-calorie diets.

Disuse of the muscles through long-term inactivity will also lead to atrophy (reduction in density) and possibly physical and mental illness.

Weight training is successfully being used to prevent and/or relieve the symptoms of osteoporosis (weakening of the bones) by firming the muscles around the bones to support the bones more efficiently.

Lifting weights doesn't necessarily turn you into Arnold Schwarzenegger. Weight training can be used to simply tone and firm the muscles without bulking-up.

The weight you use, your progressive program over time and how you lift the weights all can be tailored to suit your long-term goals and requirements.

If you have any injuries, seek the advice of a Doctor who can refer you to a qualified physiotherapist, to help your rehabilitation after sufficient rest (which is important to recharge the body and repair cells).

Sweating during exercise is normal. Sweating regularly during moderate or intense exercise, helps your body to have a more efficient water-balance system, as long as you keep hydrated with water.

WARM-UP > DYNAMIC STRETCH > MAIN ROUTINE or ROUTE > COOL-DOWN > STRETCH > RELAX…

HYDRATE & EAT

ALWAYS Warm-up by increasing intensity of effort gradually for at least 4-5 minutes, depending on intensity and duration of the main component of your routine; either cardio or weight training activities (e.g. Shorter, faster routes / races / sessions, require a longer warm-up. For longer routes such as a half marathon, conserve your energy and build up pace progressively and gradually).

Warm-up is VERY IMPORTANT for preparing the body's metabolism, and enhances the appropriate chemical reactions in the brain, to be ready for exercise.

Synovial Fluid: A good warm-up also promotes Synovial Fluid production in the joints, which keeps you supple and less likely to experience injury.

Dynamic Stretching: IMMEDIATELY after warm-up, perform dynamic stretching (or static stretching) for 10-12 seconds per muscle group, bearing in mind you need to keep your body and mind prepared for your main routine.

There is evidence to suggest that static stretching after a warm-up and before your main routine, may be contraindicated and possibly even cause injury. Dynamic stretching after warm-up is becoming more popular.

Cool-down: AFTER THE MAIN COMPONENT of your routine, ALWAYS COOL-DOWN. Cool-down gradually for 10-15 minutes after running a half marathon, or doing a triathlon. For most people 5 minutes of a cool-down should be enough. Cool-down should be a GRADUAL DECREASE of intensity and effort. Cooling the body down gradually after exercise, helps to prevent blood pooling, brings the body back to a more relaxed state and prevents injury.

STATIC STRETCH IMMEDIATELY AFTER COOL-DOWN taking at least 30 seconds for each muscle group and preferably on a mat on the floor.

Delayed Onset Muscle Soreness (DOMS): Stretching after cooldown reduces muscle soreness and increases ROM (Range of Movement) and helps you to relax. Stretching should NEVER BE PAINFUL; ease into and out of each stretch and NEVER BOUNCE.

……Take slow deep breaths and …..relax……

Proprioceptive Neuromuscular Facilitation

PNF (or Facilitated Stretching) can be very effective in increasing ROM and enhancing performance, PLEASE get advice and training in this with a qualified Fitness Trainer / Physiotherapist, or buy a book about it and read carefully BEFORE YOU ATTEMPT PNF.

During your routine be aware of:

*Your posture and correct it if necessary.

*Your core abdominal muscles should be engaged

*DO NOT lock your knees

*These checks are also useful when weight training, as is checking your form in the mirror whilst you perform your routine.

*BE AWARE of what your foot placement is like (i.e. is it to one side? This is especially important in walking and running as ideally your footfall should be a mid-foot landing roll to toe form, however try to run with your natural technique, your body will ease into a form that suits you personally.)

If you join a running club, they will also be able to help you with hints and tips on how to improve your running and training. There are also great books about running that you can buy. Also read the following chapter in this book for some hints and tips on how to enjoy running.

Some people are unaware that their feet may be supinating or pronating whilst walking or running, i.e. on either edge of the foot.

Your gait can be determined for free in many running equipment shops, to establish which trainers are more appropriate for you, but be aware the most expensive are not always the best.

I personally have found that trainers with a gap in the instep to help with flexibility of movement, a position further in for lace up and with good traction on the sole, are best for me.

I have heard mixed reactions to using orthotic insoles, so be aware that these can be expensive if not provided by the NHS and are not always necessary.

It is useful to strengthen your ankle muscles and all the complementary muscles in your legs and core-stabliser muscles, it's also useful to stretch your feet and toes gently within your Range of Movement.

Proprioception: Regular training on a safe risk-assessed surface in your bare feet, develops the proprioceptive response (muscle stabliser balance) and enhances turning and reaction speeds, as it makes the feet wider and toes more splayed.

Running and interval training

When running or walking: Move your arms in a strong full motion, check your stride, try to alter your breathing according to effort and intensity.

If you want to start running, walk more first, building up from a brisk walk… to a jog …then back to a walk …then a jog and when you are ready to speed it up, try this interval training technique to boost your endurance level: WALK > JOG > RUN > JOG > WALK > JOG > RUN > JOG > WALK etc.

You could try initially 30 seconds for each stage and increase the time for each stage as you improve. Use a stopwatch, timer or fitness app like Couch to 5k for example.

Make sure when you are walking and jogging you get to feel your ability at that moment in time, don't jog to the point where you can't run, keep each stage at a comfortable pace, and if you are really struggling for breath, slow it down, and make sure your breathing becomes steadier and more controlled.

You will know when it's time to increase your pace, and your ability to go faster for longer, and you will also know when it's best to slow it down a little, to make sure you have the energy to continue further.

Interval training is varying the speed of your effort within your ability, in a controlled way to increase endurance; this can be applied to many sports. If you would like to know more, research the various Interval Training techniques such as FARTLEK Training.

Push yourself, but if you feel dizzy or sick or sore, take it down slowly to a stop and have a few days rest before you try again.

Pushing yourself is all well and good but doesn't make sense if you are not enjoying what you are doing, and you are at risk of injuring yourself.

Time yourself and keep a record of your times, safely use visible markers like lampposts along the pavement, to make it easier to start with for running or cycling, and visible markers in the pool for swimming.

This will also give you a marker to aim for, to boost you and encourage you to begin with.

Be aware that always running on hard surfaces may affect your joints and cause shin splints, try finding outdoor tracks to run on where you know the route well and / or use a treadmill at your local gym. Treadmills are great because you can alter the speed and gradient you train on.

There are many charity events that will be fun to take part in and give you a goal to train towards, give yourself enough time to train before you attempt one of these. Bear in mind, it can take over a year to train sensibly for a marathon if you are starting from scratch. Good proper running socks are expensive but great to increase comfort and reduce the chance of getting blisters.

Find out if there are any sports clubs, walking or running groups near where you stay, as they will often know good training programs for races and charity events using the correct long-term goal training plans. The social aspect of joining an activity group is also extremely useful.

There are also a lot of great apps for your mobile phone and fitness devices to help you achieve your fitness goals.

Tips for weight training

To tone or strengthen your muscles

Before your main routine you should follow the guidelines mentioned previously for warm-up and stretch, to prepare the body and mind for weight training, prevent injury and increase performance.

Rest in between sets is VERY important to encourage recovery, enhance performance and prevent injury. This can be between 30 seconds and 3 minutes, depending on what your goals are (e.g. Hypertrophy /Endurance /Strength), and if you are a beginner, intermediate or advanced. Use a stopwatch.

Beginners workouts: Aim for 1-3 sets of 12-15 reps with 30-45 seconds rest between sets.

Once you can lift or pull or push 15 reps easily, only increase the weight when you are ready adding 2.5-5kg so that you are able to lift only within the 12-15 rep range again. Vary your routine for 12 weeks before re-assessment of the weights you are using. Alternate the upper and lower body areas in a circuit and rest for 2-3 minutes between each different exercise.

Give yourself 48 hours at least between training each area, to allow the muscles to repair. This type of low-weight training can be done once or twice a week, as a continuous on-going form of training, to maintain the tone of your muscles rather than bulking them.

If you do want to add muscle bulk, you can progress to the Intermediate level, after discussing your long-term goals with a qualified gym instructor.

Intermediate level workouts: Aim for 2-3 sets of 8-12 reps with 60-90 seconds rest between sets and 2-3 minutes between each different exercise. Vary your routine for 3 months before re-assessment of the weights you are using, adding 2.5-5kg to train in the 8-12 reps range again. As the weights and intensity have been increased you will need to rest each area even more, so train each body area only once a week.

Advanced workouts should only be started once you can lift or pull or push 12 reps easily, only increase the weight when you are ready, adding 2.5-5kg so that you are able to lift only within the 8-12 rep range again. Count to 2 seconds up, 3 seconds down. For advanced workouts, the strength trainer Anita Bean suggests: "Eight sets for legs, upper back, chest & shoulders, four sets for biceps, triceps, calves and lower back.

Rest for 3 minutes between sets, and 3-4 minutes between each different exercise. Each body part should be trained just once a week to allow recovery between workouts and muscle fibre repair".

The pain you feel after a tough workout, is a mixture of tiny tears in the muscle fibres due to exertion, and lactic acid build up.

A proper cool-down for 4 minutes gradually decreasing intensity, then stretching after a workout, helps to alleviate the pain and prevents injury. When these tears heal, that is what helps to create muscle tone and bulk; but be aware that intense pain can indicate injury, so rest, and seek medical advice.

Even Olympic Athletes experience muscle soreness after a tough workout, so don't feel that you are any less than they are. They will have trained for many years using sensible progressive, long-term program goals, broken down into shorter-term smaller goals, all developed by professional trainers.

They will have trained within their continually developing comfort zone.

If you train following a proper, sensible long-term program, you are more likely to enjoy it, keep going back and less likely to get injured so you will eventually get better results. Don't be scared to ask your gym trainer to update your program to keep it fun, interesting and fresh to encourage life-long adherence to an active lifestyle.

The number of repetitions and sets is dependent on your goals for fitness e.g. Toning, endurance, strength or bulk. 1 to 3 warm-up sets with lighter weights to prepare the muscles for using heavier weights in the following sets, is mainly used by those wanting to bulk up and / or increase strength.

It is also sensible for bodybuilders to follow a basic cardio warm-up for 4 minutes then > dynamic stretch > main weights routine > cardio cool-down for 4 minutes then > stretch on a mat, as explained before.

DO NOT HOLD YOUR BREATH. Always BREATHE OUT ON EXERTION this enhances performance, that's why the big guys make so much noise when they train, why many tennis players grunt when they hit the ball, and why martial arts fighters make a sound as they exhale when they punch and kick. Breathing out on exertion also reduces the pressure in the brain and makes lifting weights safer.

DO NOT COMPROMISE PROPER TECHNIQUE FOR HEAVIER LIFTING AS THIS CAN CAUSE INJURY!!!

To promote adherence to any weights routine, ask your gym's fitness trainer to help you find fun, interesting alternatives to the techniques you are doing to keep your routine varied and exciting. Try body-weight exercises for example, either as an alternative to the weights you are using or as a complement to your current routine, depending on your fitness level and ability.

Body-weight exercises such as burpees, lunges, squats, push-ups, pull-ups etc. can add an extra dimension to your workout and can be developed to enhance progression by adding weights, or more sets and reps.

There are different levels of great body-weight exercises to suit most abilities that can be modified as time goes on, and you become stronger and more adept at them.

E.g. For beginners push-ups you can start on your knees on a mat, and follow the instructions of a qualified instructor to keep your technique safe and appropriate. For advanced technique, you can ask your trainer to show you how to do clap push-ups; only if you can already do 40 standard push-ups easily.

Body-weight exercises are also great because you can do them at home, with little or no equipment needed.

You should always follow the guidelines mentioned previously for warm-up and stretch, then routine, cool-down and stretch, even if you are working out at home, this prevents injury and encourages enjoyment and adherence. Going up and down your stairs for 4 minutes at a gradual progressive pace, is a great way to warm-up at home.

Rest from your exercise routine is **VERY important** to encourage recovery, repair muscle fibres, enhance performance and prevent injury, so rest should be strictly scheduled into your routine program. Try to have at least 2 rest days a week, and schedule 1 or 2 weeks off your fitness training every 3 months.

More tips to increase muscle tone

I went to dance school and did lots of outdoor activities from the age of 4, so I was toned and strong by the time I was in my mid-teens.

When I started hill running, climbing, kayaking and mountain biking in my early 20's, my muscles really started to increase in bulk, strength, tone and endurance.

So, I can honestly say that from my experience, varying your activities and training program, can and will encourage all the stabiliser muscles to work and bulk up.

If you want to increase the size of your leg muscles, yes there are specific routines and workouts in the gym, BUT it would be great to also do outdoor activities, to enhance your cardiovascular fitness, as well as bulking up all the wee stabiliser muscles, as I mentioned before.

Consider varying your training routine and after a few weeks / couple of months you will notice a difference, as this will freshen up your routine, and keep you interested in adhering to exercise, at the same time as increasing muscle tone, bulk and endurance.

Outdoor activities are also great for adding a different aspect to your training, mental health is also improved just by being outside in the fresh air and sunlight.

There are so many outdoor activities for you to try, and if you have never done any of them before, always get proper instruction from a qualified instructor to keep you safe, and help you enjoy it more. Kayaking is great for core-strength and conditioning; it also works your back and arms.

Climbing and bouldering are great for all over body training. Most climbing should utilise your feet and legs for pushing up, rather than solely relying on your arms to pull you up.

When you have graduated onto including overhangs or high-grade climbs, you will use your arm and back muscles more.

There are many indoor climbing walls around the country that you can book-in with an instructor if you are a beginner. There are also lots of outdoor climbing clubs you can research.

Mountain biking is great fun and fantastic for bulking and toning your legs. Make sure that when you buy your first mountain bike, that you know how to maintain it well, get the right accessories and read up on what to take with you on long routes. Do your own research into what outdoor activities are available in your area.

Brisk walking and hill walking are fantastic hobbies to get you out into the fresh air in scenic areas, there are many rambling and hill walking groups you can research to find in your area.

The physical and mental health benefits of walking are amazing, be sure to research your route thoroughly before you go, and make sure you take all the necessary equipment e.g. map and compass, GPS, snacks, water, waterproof clothing, correct footwear, proper walking socks, first aid kit etc.

National Health Service recommendations

For people aged 18 – 64:

150 minutes (2 hours and 30 minutes) of moderate intensity aerobic activity such as cycling or fast walking every week, and muscle strengthening activities on two or more days a week that work all major muscle groups (legs, hips, back, abdomen, chest, shoulders and arms).

OR

75 minutes (1 hour and 15 minutes) of vigorous intensity aerobic activity such as running or a game of singles tennis every week, and muscle-strengthening activities on two or more days a week that work all major muscle groups (legs, hips, back, abdomen, chest, shoulders and arms).

OR

An equivalent mix of moderate and vigorous-intensity aerobic activity every week (for example two 30-minute runs plus 30 minutes of fast walking), and muscle-strengthening activities on two or more days a week that work all major muscle groups (legs, hips, back, abdomen, chest, shoulders and arms).

Physical activity for adults aged 65 and over

Older adults aged 65 or older, should ask their doctor about these recommendations taken from the NHS CHOICES website:

"If you are generally fit and have no health conditions that limit your mobility, try to be active daily and do:

At least 150 minutes (2 hours and 30 minutes) of moderate-intensity aerobic activity such as cycling or fast walking every week, and muscle-strengthening activities on 2 or more days a week that work all major muscle groups (legs, hips, back, abdomen, chest, shoulders and arms).

OR

75 minutes (1 hour and 15 minutes) of vigorous-intensity aerobic activity such as running or a game of singles tennis every week, and muscle-strengthening activities on 2 or more days a week that work all major muscle groups (legs, hips, back, abdomen, chest, shoulders and arms).

OR

An equivalent mix of moderate and vigorous-intensity aerobic activity every week (for example two 30-minute runs plus 30 minutes of fast walking), and muscle-strengthening activities on 2 or more days a week that work all major muscle groups (legs, hips, back, abdomen, chest, shoulders and arms)."

More Reasons to be active & eat well

As I mentioned earlier, light weight training is successfully being used to rehabilitate people who have *osteoporosis*, it can also help to prevent this condition, as it strengthens the muscles supporting the body's bones. Another good reason to keep reasonably active into older age, is to promote the blood flow to the extremities, which includes the brain. Your body's blood contains the oxygen, nutrients and bug-fighting cells needed to keep physically and mentally well.

Getting your posture, neck and spine checked for good alignment, can help you to see if you need to fix your posture, to keep the oxygen and nutrients flowing around your body and brain properly.

A physiotherapist can help with this assessment, and help you with exercises to correct your posture, if necessary.

Studies have found that many older people are prone to deteriorating health because they "slow down" too much after they retire, and spend too much time indoors, which not only means they are not getting enough gentle exercise, but it also means that they are getting less sunlight to their skin.

Natural sunlight helps the body to produce Vitamin D, which improves your mood, and has a role in the body's immune system efficiency, along with Vitamin C, phospholipids, and many other natural nutrients from good food.

The immune system is mainly situated in the gut; convenience food that is microwaved, apparently loses many of its nutrients in the microwaving process, which may cause you to be hungry more often, because you are not getting all the nutrients you need. It is so important to keep reasonably active, and eat as much naturally prepared food as possible, to keep healthy and happy into older age.

Much of the older generation would have grown up with good home-cooked food and were probably more active than many kids are today, when they were growing-up.

ALWAYS ask for advice from a GP AND fitness professional / physiotherapist / activity instructor BEFORE you do a new activity or sport or change your nutrition intake.

If you are pregnant or have just had a baby, ASK YOUR DOCTOR when it is safe to exercise, as the body must heal after giving birth before starting training again.

Checklist 2: Re-write this table and tick each box after reading the contents to help you understand the main points of this section and help you to set your goals.

	Speak to your Doctor before starting a new fitness and nutrition routine.
	Set long-term goals with shorter term goals, to build up gradually, sensibly and progressively.
	ALWAYS warm-up and dynamic stretch BEFORE any activity, then cool-down and stretch afterwards.
	You can get an exercise program for the gym to suit your personal goals, ask your gym instructor.
	Keep your interest in being active by varying activities and different sports and train within your comfort zone.
	I have read and understood the NHS guidelines for exercise.
	REST WHEN YOU NEED TO.

More tips for good mental health

*Make sure you get as much sleep as you need even if that means naps during the day, but be aware this might affect your night-time sleep pattern.

*Mindfulness (engaging all of the senses "in the now") and slow, deep breathing relaxation techniques. Ask your Doctor about this.

*Positive distraction e.g. exercise, listening to music on the radio, watching TV, housework, cooking, chatting to friends and family, reading, gardening, baking sweet treats.

*Ask your Doctor how to use Grounding Techniques.

*Counselling /Talking Therapy, e.g. Cognitive Behavioral Therapy. Your Doctor can refer you to a professional practitioner.

*Using accredited Mental Health Crisis services.

*Self-defense classes / Martial Arts / dance classes / art therapy / music therapy / Yoga / creative writing / voluntary work.

*Daily personal hygiene / warm bath or shower / brushing teeth. If you feel you can't have a shower or a bath, try just gently washing your face and hands in just-warm water and brushing your teeth.

If this also feels like too much, talk about what's going on for you with someone you know well and trust.

*Aromatherapy massage (which is available free, or by a small donation from some accredited health services).

*Active meditation and core-dynamics, which encourages natural anger and emotion to be physically expressed in a more positive, non-hurtful way, using pillows or cushions.

*Rest and sleep when you are tired

*Insomnia, stress, agitation, anxiety and depression can be caused by lack of exercise, or lack of sleep, lack of regular healthy nutrition / hydration and the roller-coaster ride that is life!

*Believe in the fact that YOU are the expert in your own life experiences and accept that you MAY need guidance towards recovery.

*Be open to positive healthy experiences, if you feel you are spiraling into unpleasant negativity, talk to people you know well and trust.

Visualisation techniques of what you'd like to do or a memory of somewhere nice you have been, can help when trying to sleep and on waking to encourage a better experience of the hypnagogia states (transition states between sleep and wakening)

For example: …It is a warm Spring day with a slightly cool breeze, perfect weather for going hill walking, so you dress appropriately in comfortable loose clothing and wear comfortable shoes, taking a small light rucksack with some healthy sandwiches….

….a small bag of dried fruit and nuts or oatcakes, a bottle of water and a flask of hot sweet tea….

….you get the bus with a friend you know well or a support worker to Flotterstone at the base of the Pentland Hills and start walking slowly…..

….past the Inn…along the track…you can hear the leaves on the trees rustling and smell the gorse….

…..you stroll past the field of sheep and an elderly couple walking their Sheltie dog….the sun is warm and the breeze is just the right temperature to keep you from getting too hot….

….you continue walking at a comfortable and energising pace up the wee hill to the left….

….past the cottage at the start of Glencourse reservoir that has the doves on the roof…past Kirkton Farm to the end of the reservoir opposite the field where the horses are grazing…

…you sit on the grass beside the stream…which is gently flowing over small rocks and making gurgling noises, you feel warm, relaxed and happy…

….you are ready to eat your sandwiches and drink some of your water and flask of tea…as you are sitting, a heron flies past and you follow it with your gaze taking in the beautiful scenery…..

…..then you both head back to the Inn to sit in the garden eat a scone and have a cup of tea…you get back on the bus and head home feeling relaxed and happy and ready to unwind for the evening….

Visualisation can also be useful to encourage you into doing a positive activity; see yourself doing something fun and interesting in your mind. Imagine what it would be like, or remember positive experiences of enjoyable times, as if you were doing it again in your mind. This may help you to feel what it was like and give you the motivation to seek those positive emotions again.

Motivation techniques

Everyone experiences phases where their motivation is great, and phases when it is not so good. If you can, try to determine what "inner thought voice style" motivates you personally. I had a strict "inner thought voice style" way of thinking for many years, which was incredibly stressful, but on occasion it did work to get me motivated.

Now I am a lot kinder to myself and get motivated more by kind self-talk and kind, positive thoughts. What motivates you?

Really listen to the way your mind works, if you find it very troubling, talk to someone you know well and trust and speak to your doctor who can really help you.

If the way you think about yourself and how you motivate yourself, makes you feel encouraged, brilliant, go with it. You can change the way you "thought talk" to yourself, when you realise how you currently do it, and by being determined and positive that you CAN be kind to yourself.

My Mum often quotes that shampoo advert to encourage me: "Because you're worth it"!!! This pops into my head sometimes and makes me smile! Be your own personal trainer. Trust yourself.

In Summary

Try new foods and beverages like herbal infusions instead of coffee, try new fun sports and activities, and new creative hobbies. Do something different to keep you interested in adhering to a healthy lifestyle!!

Start off slowly, building up intensity of effort gradually over time, see your fitness training as something that is fun, when it's within your comfort zone, and maintain a varied routine with different sports and activities that you enjoy. Use sensible small goals progressing and increasing slowly over time.

Use mindfulness, visualisation and relaxation to help you sleep better. See your new interests as a means of balancing mental and physical well-being.

ENJOYMENT encourages ADHERENCE!!!

You should be proud of yourself for taking an interest in healthy nutrition and fitness, good luck, believe in yourself and most importantly **HAVE FUN** with your training!

Thanks for reading my guide!

Nicole Carter

References used

My personal insight & knowledge of being Bi-polar.

The coursework and all the resources I studied for my Fitness and Nutrition qualifications.

The experience and knowledge I acquired from working as an outdoor activities instructor, fitness class instructor and personal trainer.

The complete guide to Sports Nutrition by Anita Bean.

The complete guide to Strength Training by Anita Bean.

Dynamic Stretching by Mark Kovacs.

Facilitated Stretching by Robert E. McAtee and Jeff Charland.

Advice I've been given from qualified staff at: The Edinburgh Crisis Centre; Royal Edinburgh Psychiatric Hospital Mental Health Assessment Service, Intensive Home Treatment Team and Community Mental Health Teams; Redhall Walled Garden.

New Optimum Nutrition For the Mind by Patrick Holford.

LIVESTRONG.com

NHS Choices website

EXRX.net

The Vitamin and Mineral Counter by Jody Vassallo and Dell Stanford.

The Fat, Fibre & Carbohydrate Counter by Dell Stanford.

Author Biography

Nicole Carter was born in Edinburgh in 1975 and spent most of her childhood living in Penicuik, dancing, running, playing in mud and climbing trees. Having a Bi-polar disorder has made life "difficult but interesting", with several periods of homelessness and subsequent admissions to psychiatric hospitals.

Nicole has had several articles about her printed in newspapers, some of which aren't *entirely* accurate.

Nicole has had many jobs including; Kitchen porter, office administrator for a large pensions company, cleaner, outdoor activities instructor, aerobics class instructor and personal trainer, waitress, shop assistant, activities organiser and chair exercise instructor for the elderly, which have all greatly improved her understanding of different types of people and their needs.

She has also worked in several voluntary jobs which she found to be extremely rewarding.

Life for Nicole is much more settled now and she says, "I thrive on helping other people achieve their fitness and nutrition goals to improve their mental health."

Useful Contacts

If you are struggling to cope and need somebody to talk to, each of these phone support services are available free 24 hours a day 7 days a week 365 days a year:

Samaritans UK and Republic Of Ireland: 116 123

Or if you live in Edinburgh please contact the Edinburgh Crisis Centre: 0808 8010 414 for free confidential support.

This book is dedicated to Nicole's "fantastic and supportive family".

Thank you also to: Colinton Mains House, The Cyrenians, Venture Scotland, Redhall Walled Garden, the staff of the Royal Edinburgh Psychiatric Hospital, MHAS and Community Mental Health Teams, The Edinburgh Crisis Centre, Bethany Christian Trust and Samaritans.

5 Day Food, Mood And Energy Diary

Take short notes in your notepad using these templates, to detail what you ate, drank, your mood, energy levels and your activities, to help you better understand what you need to do to start your new routine, and remember to start off slowly and build-up your goals gradually using short-term goals towards long-term goals.

Use the info to see where you can change your unhealthy habits and routines and turn that into tools to help you start and maintain better habits and routines. BE HONEST, it'll help you to see where you can make improvements!!! You CAN do this!!

Time	Monday
7am to 10am	
10am to 1pm	
1pm to 4pm	
4pm to 7pm	
7pm to 10pm	
10pm to 3am	
3am to 7am	

Time	Tuesday
7am to 10am	
10am to 1pm	
1pm to 4pm	
4pm to 7pm	
7pm to 10pm	
10pm to 3am	
3am to 7am	

Time	Wednesday
7am to 10am	
10am to 1pm	
1pm to 4pm	
4pm to 7pm	
7pm to 10pm	
10pm to 3am	
3am to 7am	

Time	Thursday
7am to 10am	
10am to 1pm	
1pm to 4pm	
4pm to 7pm	
7pm to 10pm	
10pm to 3am	
3am to 7am	

Time	Friday
7am to 10am	
10am to 1pm	
1pm to 4pm	
4pm to 7pm	
7pm to 10pm	
10pm to 3am	
3am to 7am	

My fitness and nutrition health goals...

On this date [/   /   ] I will…

In two months, I will feel…

GO FOR IT!!!